Rosemary, the Prince of Herbs
and 30 ways to use it

More books by Evelyn Key:

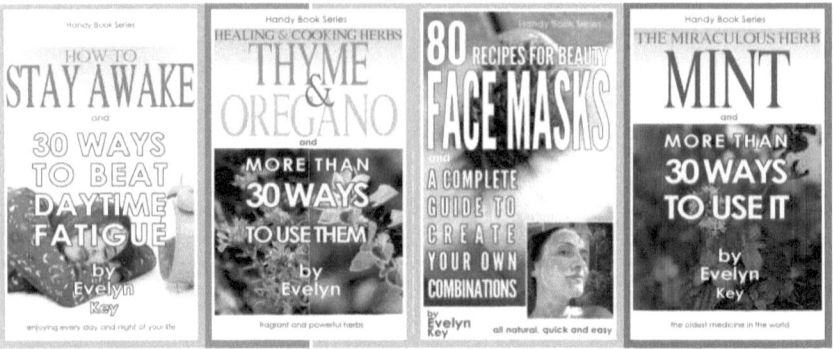

Evelyn Key

Rosemary, the Prince of Herbs
And 30 ways to use it

Evelyn Key

Handy Book Series
2014

Rosemary, the Prince of Herbs

First Printing: 2014

ISBN 978-1-312-66231-5

Evaggelia Karageorge
P.O. 1866, Agios Spyridon, Porto Rafti
Markopoulo, Attica, Greece, 19003

Handy Book Series
evelinbooks.wordpress.com
evelynbooks@gmail.com

Dedication

To all the optimist, happy and devoted people of this planet!

You create your life, you create the world!

Contents

Cautions

- Herbs are very beneficial to health, but we have to use them wisely. Large portions may cause poisoning!
- If you are pregnant, you should consult your doctor before use. In many rural areas rosemary was used for abortion.
- Symptoms of overdose include dizziness, hallucinations, convulsions and damage of the mucous membranes of the kidneys and intestines.
- During pregnancy, breastfeeding, homeopathic treatment, or if you suffer from chronic/incurable diseases, such as diabetes, cancer, cardiovascular,_hypertension, epilepsy, renal insufficiency etc, consult your doctor/physician before use.

Introduction

Rosemary, the Prince of Herbs is an introduction to the numerous uses of this wonderful, extraordinary herb: Rosemary! An herb with so many properties and benefits, variously used since ancient times until nowadays.

Following the same fun and intuitive spirit of the other books of the series, "Rosemary, the Prince of Herbs and 30 ways to use it" presents the amazing uses of rosemary through tradition, scientific facts, history and myths! Enjoy!

"Rosmarinus officinalis":

The Latin name of the herb is "Rosmarinus", meaning the "rose of the sea" because it thrives even near the sea.

According to tradition, its flowers were originally white, but their colour changed when the Virgin Mary threw her garment on the plant. The flowers turned suddenly blue. So, it was named "Rose of Mary" in her honour.

Rosemary has played a very powerful role in the Mediterranean life, both as gastronomic ingredient and a healing herb. You can use rosemary to prepare healing beverages or give your meals a special flavour, to relieve headaches, to stimulate your hair growth, even as an elixir of youth! I almost forgot: If you are a witch, be aware because it may… vanquish you... But I suppose you already know that!

Rosemary is an herb that one should definitely have in their garden.

Its flavour is intense, spicy and somewhat bitter.

Rosemary is a shrub with very small and thin leaves, densely packed on the branches, and green all year long. Its flowers are blue-purple and in some cases, white. It grows in any soil, even if it's rocky.

You can grow a rosemary bush, simply by planting sprigs from a larger plant! Remember to put the sprigs in a vase of water for 5 to 6 days before you plant them.

Rosemary, the Prince of Herbs

It is a very durable and decorative shrub while it has very few growing requirements. It can be easily adapted in your garden or balcony, as long as there is sufficient sunlight.

Rosemary doesn't like too much moisture in the soil. Over-watering may rot the root and cause even the death of the plant by fungi attack.

According to the bibliography, rosemary blooms from March to June... However, last year mine blossomed in February!

For your hair only...

Rosemary rejuvenates and **reconstructs distressed hair**. Also removes grease and it is considered as an "herbal medicine" against hair loss. This is why it is often used as a basic ingredient in many hair products.

Rinse it!
Just rinse your hair with rosemary water.

In a large bowl, add 2 tbsp of dried rosemary leaves and 1 tbsp of chamomile (1). Pour 1 quart of hot water and let it cool down.

Strain it into another container or a jug and use it after shampooing as the final rinse. Gently massage your hair, comb and let them dry.

Repeat for 5-6 shampooing for better results.

Mask it!
A mask recipe that treats your hair from the roots to the tips, while it strengthens and tones the scalp.

You need:
½ cup of olive oil
½ fresh squeezed lemon
1 egg yolk
2 tsp of dried rosemary leaves (2)

For an easier and cheaper version, use just the olive oil and the rosemary.

Preparation:
In a pot, mix the oil and the rosemary, over low heat. (3)

When the mixture gets warm, remove from fire and let it cool down.

After 20 minutes, strain, add the egg yolk and the lemon juice and mix until they get unified. Apply the mixture to your hair, massage your scalp, and let it sit for about 20 minutes.

Rosemary, the Prince of Herbs

Then, wash your hair very well.

Tip: Apply the shampoo directly on your hair and wash well with no water. The oil will be removed easier this way. Afterwards, rinse with water and shampoo (4) again.

Preparing natural cosmetics, is fun, inexpensive and enhances your beauty care ritual!

Memory improvement?

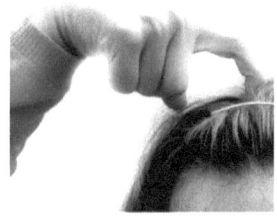

Rosemary improves **concentration and memory**.
It is considered as the ideal herb for mental fatigue.

Drink it!

Studies have shown (a) that rosemary **stimulates the synthesis of the main nerve growth factor, NGF**, a factor that prevents damage and death of the human cells.

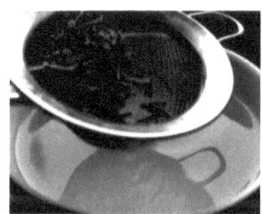

Prepare a nice cup of rosemary infusion:
Choose a rosemary twig with leaves and a few flowers, and put it in a pot. Pour 2 cups of hot water and let it stay for 7-10 minutes. Strain and serve.
Drink warm with a teaspoon of honey if desired.
Combine with orange slices or ginseng!
If you drink 1-2 cups a day for 3 weeks, then you have to take a one week break before you continue for another 3 weeks. (5)

Wear it!

Rosemary **is considered a natural memory enhancer.** It has the ability to stimulate blood circulation when it comes in contact with the body. Probably this is why the ancient Greeks used to wear garlands of rosemary on their heads in cases of hard study.

If you find it hard to fashion a rosemary garland as the ancient Greeks did, you could try something easier, such as:

Take one or two sprigs of rosemary and fasten them around your forehead with a hair ribbon.

Rosemary, the Prince of Herbs

Well, this might look a bit funny, but when the concentration and mental acuity are essentials, then it's worth a try!

Smell it!

According to <u>British researchers</u> (b), even the smell of rosemary can enhance human mental capacity.

There are many ways to enjoy the pleasure and the benefits of rosemary scent. **Here are some ideas:**

- Add 10 drops of rosemary, 6 drops of lemon and 1 drop of sage essential oils in boiling water, lean close to the pot and breathe the scented steam. If you don't have essential oils, just add a handful of dried rosemary.
- Use the same blend of essential oils, or just rosemary, in an essential oil warmer. You can also use an electric diffuser. There are many kinds available in the market, suitable even for your car!
- Sprinkle a few drops of rosemary essential oil on a cloth handkerchief, and smell it whenever you want, wherever you are!

Do you have a sunny window? Just plant rosemary in a pot, and smell it all the time!

Boost your love life!

The intense and penetrating perfume of rosemary has aphrodisiac properties.

It regulates the adrenal glands and hormone production; it warms up, stimulates and prolongs the sexual pleasure!

Spice it!

It is no coincidence that in ancient Greece, rosemary was regarded as a gift of the goddess Aphrodite (Venus)!

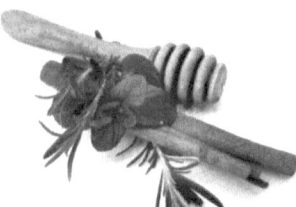

All the Olympian Gods were archetypes, associated with many symbolisms. So was Aphrodite, who symbolized the divine matchmaker and the stimulating factor of sensual desire.

Prepare a boosting infusion for special occasions:

In a pot, pour 2 cups of water, add 1 teaspoon of rosemary flowers, 1 teaspoon of peppermint leaves and 1 cinnamon stick, and bring to a boil. Remove from fire and let it stay for about 7-10 minutes.

Strain well, add 2 tsp of honey and drink very slowly.

Caution: Large quantities won't bring better results; they may cause drowsiness and dizziness instead.

Massage it!

On his honeymoon, Napoleon is said to have used hundreds of bottles of rosemary scented water! Maybe that's not just a story.

Rosemary has excellent tonic and stimulant properties, especially for cases of sexual problems caused by severe fatigue.

Prepare a massage oil blend:

In a small bottle, mix 100 ml (3.5Oz) almond oil with 20 drops of rosemary, 10 drops jasmine or rose and 10 drops of cinnamon essential oils. Blend and enjoy!

Rosemary, the Prince of Herbs

Or

Mix 20 drops of rosemary essential oil in 1 Oz (25-30ml) almond oil.

Massage the tired muscles of the body and temples. Don't forget to treat hands and feet!

Is there anything better than a relaxing massage to rejuvenate the erotic mood?

Serve it!

During the European Middle Ages, rosemary was used as an ingredient in erotic filters.

Though it might not be quite a magic potion, serving a **flavoured glass of wine** to your partner, sounds like a pleasant idea!

You need:
8 cups of red wine
2 branches of fresh rosemary
3.5 ounces sugar
1 cinnamon stick

Preparation: Put the rosemary, the cinnamon and the sugar in a container or a jar with a cap, and add the wine. Close the cap and **let it in a dark place for about 8-10 days**. Shake well once a day to dissolve the sugar. Strain the mixture and serve at room temperature.

One glass of wine each time is enough!

What is good for the heart and blood vessels, is also good for sexual health...!

Migraines or Headaches?

Infusions or decoctions of rosemary are widely used as healing beverages for headaches.

Rubbing of the forehead with rosemary oil can be very beneficial for chronic migraines.

Placing a moist fabric, dipped in water with a few drops of rosemary essential oil, on the forehead, relieves in all cases.

Compress it!

Pour 2 ½ cups of water into a bowl, add 10 drops of rosemary essential oil (6) and stir. Immerse a small towel, or any cotton fabric, into the bowl for a few minutes. Then squeeze it and place it on your forehead.

Press gently with your fingers, close your eyes and relax for a few minutes.

Repeat more than one time, if the headache is intense.

Some soft music that makes you feel happy, might also help while relaxing!

Infuse it!

Rosemary reduces the dilation of blood vessels, thereby relieves headache.

Prepare a healing infusion:
In a pot, add
1 tsp of rosemary leaves or flowers,
½ tsp of mint leaves,
½ tsp of sage leaves
Pour 2 cups of hot water.
Cover and let it stay for 10 minutes.
Strain and add 1 tsp of honey if you like.

1 cup, 2 times a day for 3-4 days in the row, is enough.

Remember that: relaxation is equally important for headache and migraine relief.

So, one more recipe with extra relaxing properties: Follow the same procedure as above, using the following ingredients this time:
3 cups of hot water
1 tbsp of rosemary leaves or flowers
1 tsp of chamomile
1 tsp of valerian
Rosemary's digestive substances, stimulate the liver and cleanse the body of toxins.

Rub it!

Rubbing the forehead, the temples and the nape with a rosemary oil mixture, can relieve **the pains of the head.**

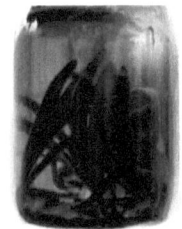

Create your own rosemary oil extract:
Use a plant oil as a base, such as almond oil.
3.5 Oz almond oil
5 tsp dried rosemary leaves
Preparation: Put the rosemary leaves in a small sterilized jar or bottle, add the almond oil and close the cap. Place it in a warm and sunny spot, for 3 weeks, and shake it once a day.

Then, drain the oil very carefully using a muslin cloth. Keep it in a dark glass bottle, in a cool and shady place.

Apply the homemade oil extract your forehead, temples and back of your neck, and massage gently.
You can use the same analogy to prepare any herbal oil extract you want.

Headaches and migraines are caused by numerous factors, such as fatigue, tension and anxiety, digestive problems, colds, allergies, etc.

So, you can use essential oils (7) to prepare a massage oil, suitable for your special condition.

Try one of the following combinations:
1 tsp of almond or sesame oil

+

- 2 drops of rosemary essential oil and 1 drop of mint essential oil. (for headaches is caused by fatigue.)
- 1 drop of rosemary, 1 drop of lavender and 1 drop of chamomile essential oils. (for tension and stress.)
- 2 drops of rosemary and 2 drops of eucalyptus essential oils. (For headaches derived from colds and allergies.)

Essential oils must be 100% pure, not adulterated or synthetic. You may consider consulting an aromatherapist for further advice.

Syrup it!

You need:
3 cups hot water
2 sprigs of rosemary
1 fresh squeezed lemon
½ cup of honey
1 pound of sugar

Prepare: In a pot, put the rosemary and the hot water. Cover and let the infusion rest for about 10 minutes.

Strain into a saucepan, add the lemon juice, the honey and the sugar and simmer over low heat. Keep stirring until sugar dissolves and the syrup thickens.

Pour into a clean, dry jar and let it cool before you close the cap.

2 tablespoons a day, for 3-4 days are enough. (1 in the morning, 1 in the evening)

Caution: Do not use any of the above mixtures **without asking your physician**: during pregnancy, breastfeeding, if you apply some homeopathic treatment, or if you suffer from chronic/incurable diseases, such as diabetes, cancer, cardiovascular,_hypertension, epilepsy, renal insufficiency etc.

Prepare Your Own Tincture

Tincture is the alcoholic extract of an herb. (Alcohol 35-90% by volume). Alcoholic ethanol solutions such as vodka or white rum (alcohol 40-50%) are often used for this purpose, as well as strong apple cider vinegar.

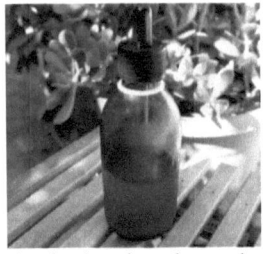

Ingredients:
A handful of dried rosemary or (1 cup of fresh)
1 cup of alcohol
Preparation: Do not use metal objects to cut the rosemary. Put in a glass or ceramic jar with a lid that closes tight; no metal parts. (8) Mash the leaves a bit with a ceramic pestle. Pour the alcohol, stir, close the jar and shake slightly.

Place it in a shady place for up to 1 month, shaking once a day or every other day. Thereafter, strain and store in a small dark glass bottle, with a dropper on the cap if possible.

The dropper is very useful, since you will be using only a few drops of this formulation.

What about beauty elixirs

There is a myth about a famous elixir of youth, which transformed the seventy years old Queen Elizabeth of Hungary into an attractive young woman. She looked so much young and beautiful, that the 25 year old King of Poland asked her hand in marriage, at 1370 AD.

The elixir was named after her, "Water of the Queen of Hungary", and it was produced by the distillation of rosemary, cedar and turpentine.

I would love to share the complete recipe, but unfortunately I don't have it! However, if you find it first, I hope you won't forget me!

Salt it!

Prepare your own rosemary bath salts:
You need:

3 tbsp of dried rosemary leaves and flowers (or 1 tbsp of rosemary, 1 tbsp of chamomile, 1 tbsp of lavender flowers)

1 cup of Sea Salt

1 cup of any Exotic Salt (Celtic, Dead Sea, Himalayan, Hawaiian)

3 tbsp sweet almond oil

3-4 drops of rosemary and orange essential oils (optional)

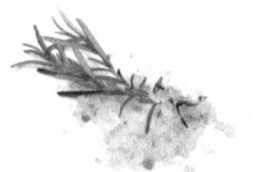

Prepare: Mash the herbs a bit with a pestle in a jar. Add the rest of the ingredients. Close the cap and let the herbs infuse their juices for at least one day (2 days is the best).
Add one handful of the salt mixture in the hot bathtub water. Enjoy!

Bathe it!

"If you are feeling weak, boil rosemary leaves in fresh water, wash yourself and then you will shine... smell it and feel young..." [Medieval literature]

<u>Bathing in rosemary is said to be a wholesome skin care.</u>

Here are two ways to prepare a rosemary bath:
In a pot, add 1 cup of rosemary leaves and 2 cups of hot water, cover it and let it stay for 20-30 minutes. Strain and keep the infusion aside.

Take a quick shower and rub your body gently with a loofah, to get rid of dead skin cells.

Then, fill the bathtub with hot water, add the rosemary infusion and enjoy a relaxing bath!

If you have some rosemary oil extract, add 1 tsp in the bathtub water!

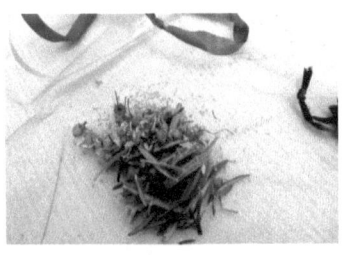

For the second option, you will need:
2 tbsp of rosemary leaves and flowers
1 tsp of chamomile and 1 tsp of lavender
(Best use fresh herbs, but if you can't find any, you can use dried).
Put the herbs in a tulle cloth and fold it to make a pouch.

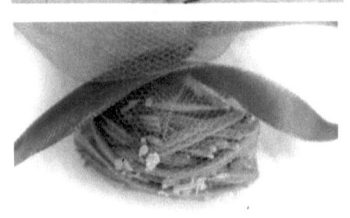

Tie it with a ribbon and plunge into the hot bath water.

Relax and enjoy your bath while the herbs infuse their beneficial substances.
Use the pouch to massage gently your body!

Add a handful of your homemade bath salts and let the joyance take you off!

Lotion it!
You need:
2 tsp of rosemary, dried leaves and flowers (or 2 tbsp of fresh leaves)
2 cups of water
Preparation: Bring the water into a boil, add the rosemary leaves and let it simmer for about 10-12 minutes. Remove from fire

and let it cool down. Strain in a small jar or bottle. You can store it in the fridge for 4-5 days.

Application: Put some lotion on a cotton pad and gently spread it on a clean face. If you have swollen eyes, press slightly the swollen spots with the cotton pad.

Next, follows and advanced lotion for skins with more complex problems such as oiliness, acne or pimples, scars and inflammation:

2 cups of water
2 tbsp of rosemary leaves and flowers
1 tsp of fresh black peppercorns
2 tsp of apple vinegar

Preparation: In a pot, add the rosemary, the pepper and the water. Bring the mixture into a boil, lower the heat and let it simmer until half of the liquid evaporates.

Remove from fire and let it cool down. Strain into a bottle, add the apple vinegar and shake well.

Apply on clean skin, right before you go to bed at night. Store in the fridge for a few days.

These three ingredients have powerful properties, such as:
Antioxidant, antiseptic (rosemary)
Antibacterial (pepper)
Vitamins A and C (apple vinegar)

A few drops of rosemary tincture, can make these lotions even more effective.

History And Myths

In the ancient Greek language, the name of rosemary was "Livanotis". Combined with frankincense, myrrh and other herbs it was used as incense for ritual cleansings.

In many places, rosemary was believed to be a symbol of the birth of Christ.

It is also said that it was one of the herbs that God gave the first human beings, when they were expelled from Paradise. This is why this herb has so special healing powers; it is its purpose to relieve mankind.

According to astrologers, rosemary is the herb of the Sun.

The ancient Greeks and Romans appreciated it very much. They used to burn it as incense next to the altars, so to please the gods and hear their prayers. As maintained by the ancient Greek Mythology, the goddess Aphrodite gifted rosemary to the humans.

Repel poisonous animals and insects

"If you put the leaves at the door and at two or three other places in your house, snakes will not hurt you, neither scorpions nor any other poisonous animals. Even if there is a snake in a hole, burn some rosemary there next to it. Feeling the smell, the snake exits to go away or dies..."

This is what says Agapios, a monk from Crete Island, in his book "Geoponikon", written back in 1634 AD.

Spread it!

You can spread rosemary leaves in front of your doors and windows. You could also hang little bags with dried leaves; try to hang them as close to the ground as possible.

Of course, if there is enough space and sunlight, plant some rosemary shrubs in pots and let them guard your doors and windows.

Spray it!

Prepare your own spray repellent:

In 2 cups of boiling water, add 1 cup of chopped rosemary and 1 mashed garlic clove, and cover. Remove from fire and let it stay for about 2 hours.

Then strain the liquid into a vaporizer.

Spray the passages through where the reptiles and insects enter your home.

You can make it stronger, by adding 1 tbsp Melissa and 1 tbsp Mint leaves.

Protect your clothes from moths: Place little bags of thin cloth in your closets, filled with a mixture of rosemary, sage, lavender and basil.

Gathering And Storing

Gather whole, small tender branches. The best time to collect is early in the morning or in the afternoon.

Then, you have to desiccate and store: Pluck the leaves on a cotton towel. Put it in a cool and dry place away from the sun. When dried, keep them in a clean and dry jar and cover.

However, you can find very good quality packaged rosemary.

Let's do some cooking!

It is true that in the gastronomy area, rosemary has been mostly used as a flavouring for meats, poultry and fish.

For example, in Italy they use it with lamb, beef, rabbit, chicken and fish, but they also include it in pasta sauces, breads, pizzas and desserts recipes.

In France is a well known flavouring for some kinds of ham, and some tonic wines.

On Crete island, rosemary is called "Arismari" and it is very popular in snail dishes.

As a vegetarian myself, I will give you two meatless recipes below:

Potato it!

How about some Baked Potatoes with rosemary?

Serves 2. Preparation and cooking time: 50-60 minutes

Ingredients

1 pound of small round potatoes (organic)

½ cup of olive oil

1 tbsp mustard

1 tsp sugar

3 tsp white wine

½ cup of rosemary leaves

1 tsp red pepper (cayenne)

1 freshly squeezed lemon

½ cup of water

Salt and pepper

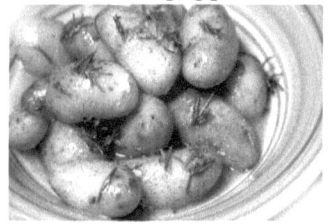

Preparation: Scrub and wash the potatoes very well, with the peel. Boil them for about 10 minutes. Strain and put them in an oven proof dish.

In a blender, add the olive oil, the mustard, the sugar, the wine, the red pepper, the lemon juice, the water, salt and pepper.

Blend until the mixture becomes creamy, and then pour over the potatoes.

Add about ½ cup of water.

Sprinkle with the rosemary leaves, mix and bake in preheated oven at 180 °C (356°F), on the bottom grate for about 25-30 minutes.

Serve with a fine glass of chilled white wine!

Bean it!

Rosemary is a great flavouring also for foods cooked with wine or garlic.

Preparation and cooking time: 20 minutes

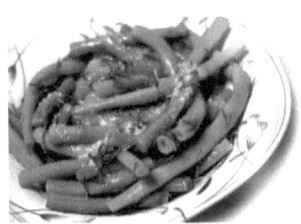

Ingredients

2 pounds of round green beans (fresh or frozen)

1 tsp of rosemary (dried or fresh)

1 tsp of salt

¼ cup of vinegar

½ cup of olive oil

1 crushed or finely chopped garlic clove (optional)

Preparation: Pour half a gallon (2 Lt) of water in a kettle, add the rosemary and the salt and bring to a boil. Then, toss in the beans and cook for about 15 minutes, until they get tender. Strain and keep aside.

Mix well the oil with the vinegar and the garlic, add a little salt and pour over the beans!

Enjoy as a side dish or a salad!

Flavour your salad!

Rosemary is a superb ingredient for condiment oils, vinegars and cooking salts.

Oil it!

A flavoured oil that matches wonderfully with salads, baked potatoes, eggplants and mushrooms, grilled meats, poultry and fish.

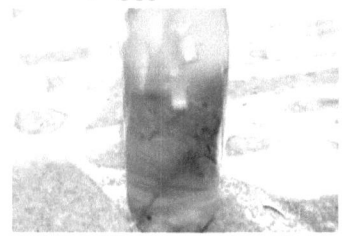

You need:
4 cups (about 1lt) of extra virgin olive oil
2 twigs of rosemary
2 garlic cloves
1 tsp of pink and black peppercorns
1 lemon slice

Preparation: Wash the rosemary twigs, peel the garlic cloves and cut them in half. Put all the ingredients in a bottle, pour the olive oil and close the cap.

Keep it in a shady and cool place, for at least 2 weeks, before it's ready to season your dishes!

Olive oil with rosemary can be easily combined with other flavours and aromas.

Vinegar it!

During the European Middle Ages, there was a vinegar mixed with herbs, that was believed to banish the plague: The "four thieves vinegar", and rosemary was one of its ingredients.

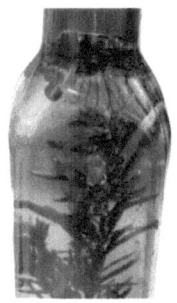

However, next follows a vinegar for salads!
You need:
2 cups of vinegar
1 sprig of fresh rosemary
1 tsp of red-green-white and black peppercorns
1 dark glass bottle

Preparation: Put the rosemary and the peppercorns in the bottle.

Fill the bottle with vinegar and close well.
Store it in a cool, dark place for 3 weeks.

Rosemary, the Prince of Herbs

Then, strain, or leave the ingredients inside the bottle and use a small strainer every time you serve.

Enjoy it in your salads!

Clean the air and feel good

Long ago, people used to burn rosemary in hospitals to disinfect the air.

Actually, this practice still exists, at least until a few years ago, in some French hospitals, where they burn rosemary along with cedar nuts.

Diffuse it!

In the 14th century, the plague epidemic killed thousands human beings. As a way of protection, people carried in their clothes punches of rosemary, to inhale it when they were passing through infected places.

You can buy a diffuser and use rosemary essential oil.

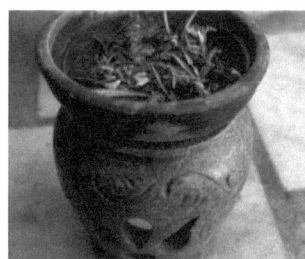 However, there are alternative ways to diffuse rosemary's disinfectant properties, more convenient and economical.

All you need is classic ceramic oil warmer. Put a little water in the dish and fill it with rosemary leaves. Light the candle and you're done! For best results, let the leaves in the water for 1-2 hours before you light the candle.

If you have already made a rosemary oil extract, add a tsp in the water!

Apply this idea to scent your space with any natural herb and spice you like, such as vanilla, cinnamon, lavender etc.

Burn it!

Do you have a fireplace? Great! Throw a few rosemary twigs in the fire and let the natural scent of the burning leaves fill the room!

Dried herbs can be perfectly used as a natural tinder!

By burning rosemary in your fireplace, you also help in the disinfection of the city air.

Steam it!

In a pot, pour 3 cups of water. Add 2 twigs of rosemary and bring to a boil. As it boils, bring the pot into the centre of the room you want to refresh.

Don't forget to place it on a heat resistant pad.

Alternatively, instead of rosemary twigs you can add 6-8 drops of rosemary essential oil.

If it is winter, you can place the pot on a radiator, to extend the steaming.

Banish negative energy

As I said before, during the European Middle Ages, people believed that rosemary grows in the yards of ethical people!

They also believed that it brings good luck and protects from witches and evil spirits.

Plant it!

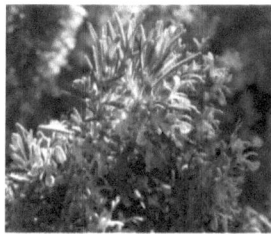

Rosemary grows in any soil, even if it is rocky. You can grow a new rosemary bush, simply by planting sprigs from a larger plant!

Before planting, put the sprigs in the water for 5 to 6 days. Then plant them directly in the ground or in pots.

It is a very durable and decorative shrub with very few growing requirements. It can be easily adapted in your garden or balcony, as long as there is sufficient sunlight.

Incense it!

Follow the ancient rituals and burn rosemary as an incense.

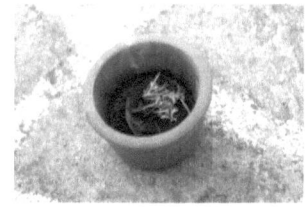

In an incense burner or a small ceramic bowl, place a charcoal tablet and burn it.

Put 1 tsp of dried rosemary on top of the charcoal, and let the scent of burning leaves purify the space.

Enhance the cleansing effect, by adding a few sage leaves!

Step on it!

Put rosemary under the front door mat!

This way, every time you, or a visitor, step on it, negative energies will be "captured" at the entrance and won't even cross the doorway!

History And Myths

Another legend about rosemary, narrates the story of Lebanon, an excellent young man who was dedicated to the gods. Unfortunately, Lebanon was murdered by disrespectful people. Then, Goddess Earth transformed him into an aromatic bush so he could honour the gods with his fragrance.

During the European Middle Ages, rosemary, was grown in every garden. People back then believed that rosemary thrived in the yards of the righteous people! It was also believed to give good luck and protect from witches and evil spirits.

The ability of rosemary to enhance memory, turned it into a symbol of fidelity, friendship and reminiscences.

Soothe your intensine – Lift up your energy

"Boil rosemary flowers in water, until the half is left, and drink the water. That will heal any illness you have in your intestines.." (Monk Agapios "Geoponikon")

Cocktail it!
A nice cool herb & juice cocktail!

You need:
1 cup of water
1 tbsp of dried rosemary
1 cup of pomegranate juice
1 tsp of honey or agave syrup (optional)
Preparation: Boil the dried rosemary in the water for 5-6 minutes. Remove from heat, add the honey or syrup, stir and let it cool down. Strain in a pot, add the pomegranate juice, stir and serve in a glass!

Mix it!
Rosemary is considered an excellent body tonic. Combined with other tonic herbs, provides a powerful energy drink!
You need:
1 tsp of dried rosemary
½ tsp of ginseng
½ tsp of licorice root
3 cups of water
Put the three herbs in a pot and pour hot water over them. Cover the pot and let it stay for 10 minutes. Add 2-3 tsp of honey if desired.

Serve hot or, when it cools down, put it in the fridge and serve later, with ice cubes and an orange slice.

Ginseng belongs to the leader team of tonic herbs. Licorice increases the healing properties and reduces the bitter taste of the other herbs.

Some Rosemary Benefits

- <u>Recent studies</u> (b) show that rosemary can protect the brain from stroke, neurodegeneration and Alzheimer's disease.
- Ideal for mental fatigue
- Cardiotonic
- Regulates the adrenal glands
- Cholagogue
- Expectorant
- Lung antiseptic (bronchitis, influenza, whooping cough, asthma)
- Helps intestinal disorders (colitis, diarrhoea, gas)
- Digestive
- Tonic for vision
- Stimulates the nervous system
- Good for rheumatism and muscle aches
- For sprains and bruises
- The gargling is good for oral ulcers
- The juice of mashed fresh rosemary leaves, stops alopecia.

Sweet Dreams!

"Put the leaves under your pillow so not to see bad dreams.." As monk Agapios says in "Geoponikon"

Pillow it!

Traditionally, rosemary was used for a good and deep night's sleep and to keep away bad dreams.

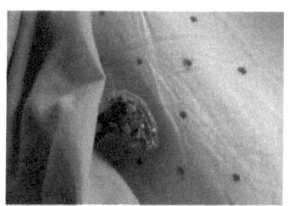

Simple as that:

Apply a practice that dates back centuries: Put some rosemary leaves and flowers in a small bag and place it under your pillow. Have sweet dreams!

Make a small pillow filled with rosemary, and lay your head every tie you want to have a peaceful sleep with nice and vivid dreams, or even just relax.

A long time ago, young girls used to put rosemary under their pillows, so to dream of the love of their life.

But most of all:
Enjoy it!
Thank you!

Notes

1. *(Rinse your hair with rosemary):* If your hair is blond, use 2 tbsp of chamomile and 1tbsp of rosemary.

2. *(Hair mask recipe):* If you have blond hair, add 1 tsp of chamomile and 1 tsp of rosemary.

3. *(Hair mask recipe):* Be careful, keep the fire low not to burn the oil.

4. *(Hair mask recipe):* Always use mild, organic shampoos.

5. *(Herbal infusions):* Do not take the same herb for periods longer than 2-3 months.

6. *(Rosemary Compress)* instead of essential oil you can add a few drops of your rosemary oil extract or tincture.

7. *(Essential Oils):* Always use essential oils diluted and never directly to the skin.

8. *(Tincture):* Metals and plastic materials can cause unwanted reactions in contact with alcohol, such releasing dangerous chemicals.

9. *(Cooking):* If you use large quantities, food might taste a bit of camphor.

10. *"Carnosic acid, a component of rosemary (Rosmarinus officinalis L.), promotes synthesis of nerve growth factor in T98G human glioblastoma cells.."* [Kosaka K1, Yokoi T., Biol Pharm Bull. 2003 Nov;26(11):1620-2., www.ncbi.nlm.nih.gov]

11. *"To investigate the effect that smell can have on the brain, Dr Mark Moss and his colleagues asked 144 volunteers to complete a series of long-term memory, working memory, and attention and reaction tests in a scent-free cubicle or one infused with either rosemary or lavender. Results showed that those in the rosemary-infused cubicles have better long-term memory than those in the unscented cubicles, while those in the lavender-scented cubicles performed worse on tests of working memory and reaction times."* [Rosemary May Boost Memory, WoldHealth.Net, Reported by www.reutershealth.com on the 28 March 2002]

12. *"In two expedited publications by The Journal of Neurochemistry and Nature Reviews Neuroscience, the scientists report for the first time that CA (the active ingredient in rosemary, known as carnosic acid) activates a novel signalling pathway that protects brain cells from the ravages of free radicals. In animal models, the scientific group, led by Drs. Takumi Satoh (Iwate University, Japan) and Stuart Lipton (Burnham Institute), found that CA becomes activated by the free radical damage itself, remaining innocuous unless needed, exactly what is wanted in a drug. "* [ScienceDaily, Source: Burnham Institute for Medical Research]

References

1. Contemporary Complete Treatment With Herbs, Ignatiou M. Zagharopoulou, Special agriculturalist Professor, Psichalos publications

2. 200 herbs and their healing properties, Roula Goliou – Biologist, Maliaris publications

3. Herbs and Fruits, Mirsini Labraki

4. Geoponikon, Agapios monk, 1796, The Digital Library of Modern Greek Studies

5. 100 Herbs 1000 Remedies, Kostas Bazaios

Glossary

Infusion: The extract produced by soaking the herb in hot water (or other liquid.)

Decoction: The liquid resulting from boiling the herb.

Oil extract: The herbal infusion in oil.

Tincture: The extract of an herb into consumable alcohol or other ethanol solutions, such as vodka, white rum, vinegar.

Essential oil: The natural oil, which is extracted from the herb by distillation

Disclaimer

The above information is a sharing of traditional knowledge and experiences for educational and informational purposes. It does not constitute medical diagnosis or medication recommendation. This book is not intended to substitute professional diagnosis and treatment. Also, is not intended to replace any medication you are already taking or the advice of your doctor.

The author and the publishers disclaim any warranties and are not liable for excessive and careless use, for any incidental or consequential damage connected direct or indirectly with the content of this ebook, or the ignoring of the recommendations of your doctor.

The liability, use, misuse, negligence of any recipe, instruction or ideas given in this book is under the total responsibility of the reader.

Author and publisher disclaim also any warranties for the accuracy of the external links content.

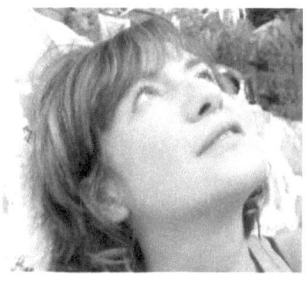

"Hello again!
I love cooking and gardening, but most of all I enjoy learning. Since I moved to the countryside, I 'm growing herbs and practicing on them, a daily routine that gives me joy and a new respect for the power of nature. When I saw the blossomed rosemary shrub in my garden this spring, the idea of writing about this magnificent herb, inspired me. I hope it will be as fun and informative for you, reading it, as it was for me, writing it! Thank you!!"

Visit : http://evelinbooks.wordpress.com

for updates, beauty and cooking recipes, tips and instructions for homemade products, ideas sharing and lots of colourful images!